W9-CHN-194

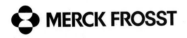

GRAHAM E. TROPE

GLAUCOMA
A Patient's Guide to the Disease

UNIVERSITY OF TORONTO PRESS
Toronto Buffalo London

© University of Toronto Press Incorporated 1997
Toronto Buffalo London
Printed in Canada

ISBN 0-8020-7847-8

Printed on acid-free paper

Canadian Cataloguing in Publication Data

Trope, Graham E.
  Glaucoma : a patient's guide to the disease
  ISBN 0-8020-7847-8
  1. Glaucoma – Popular works.   I. Title.
  RE871.T76 1996   617.7'41   C96-931484-1

University of Toronto Press acknowledges the
financial assistance to its publishing program of the
Canada Council and the Ontario Arts Council.

Publication of this book has been made
possible through a publication subsidy from
Merck Frosst Canada Inc.

This book is dedicated to all patients who have taken the time to enquire about glaucoma, to the Glaucoma Research Society of Ontario, and especially to Angela, Samantha, and Matthew.

Contents

II TESTS FOR GLAUCOMA

III ALL ABOUT TREATMENT

Isopto® Carpine is a trademark of Alcon Canada Inc.
Miocarpine™ is a trademark of CIBA Vision Ophthalmics
Phospholine Iodide® is a trademark of Storz; Division of
Wyeth Ayerst Canada Inc.

Iopidine® is a trademark of Alcon Canada Inc.
TRUSOPT® is a trademark of Merck & Co., Inc., Merck Frosst
    Canada Inc., licensed user

FIGURES

GLOSSARY OF GLAUCOMA TERMS

Preface

Glaucoma is unlike any other affliction. It usually causes no pain, discomfort, or distress. Central vision remains excellent until the very last
stages of the condition. Patients are therefore
often confused and initially reluctant to believe
their vision is in danger. The purpose of this
book is to inform patients about glaucoma, and
to provide some insight into this condition.
Information allows the patient to actively participate in the decision-making process along the
long road to successful maintenance of vision.

This book was inspired by the thoughtful
questions I've been asked by numerous patients.
Although there are excellent textbooks on glaucoma available in many libraries, they are written primarily for eye specialists, and can be
difficult to obtain and understand for the average person. There is very little information available written in a straightforward manner for the
patient suffering from glaucoma.

This book presents information about the

major aspects of glaucoma in a simple question-and-answer style. Many of the questions are ones that I have been asked over the years. My hope is that this book will provide you, the reader, with enough information to understand the disease and to actively participate in the fight against one of humanity's major causes of blindness, glaucoma.

Thanks to Mr Stephen Gordon for the illustrations in this book, and to Carol Goldhar for preparing the manuscript.

All about Glaucoma

1 / What is glaucoma?

Chronic open-angle glaucoma (also known as primary open-angle glaucoma) is a painless condition, usually associated with high pressure in the eye, which results in nerve damage and loss of vision. Normal pressure varies between 12 and 21 mmHg. Pressure is formed by fluid passing through the eye. This fluid, called the aqueous humour, is produced by a gland called the ciliary processes. The aqueous humour drains out of the eye through tissue in the front of the eye called the trabecular meshwork. The increased pressure causing glaucoma occurs when fluid flow through the eye's drainage system is obstructed (see figure 1, p. 51). High pressure is not always dangerous. In susceptible individuals, however, this high pressure does damage the eye, and in particular, the nerve at the back of the eye (see figure 2, p. 52). The nerve becomes cupped and eventually the vision starts to fail. The loss of peripheral or side vision is characteristic of glaucoma. Central vision, especially in the early stages, is typically not affected.

2 / What is the difference between glaucoma and ocular hypertension?

Glaucoma refers specifically to high pressure causing damage to the optic nerve and/or the peripheral vision. Ocular hypertension refers to high pressure which does not damage the nerve or vision. Patients with ocular hypertension are often called glaucoma suspects. Most glaucoma suspects do not go on to develop glaucomatous nerve and vision damage.

3 / My doctor says I am a glaucoma suspect. What does this mean?

A glaucoma suspect is a patient with high pressure but without damage to the optic nerve or visual field. Most patients with ocular hypertension do not require treatment, and will not get glaucoma. However, about 33 per cent of patients with high pressure do eventually go on to develop glaucomatous damage. As a result it is absolutely essential that glaucoma suspects be examined at least once a year to rule out the development of early damage and the need for therapy.

4 / What is normal eye pressure?

Normal eye pressure is between 12 and 21

millimetres of mercury (mmHg), with average pressure being 15.5 mmHg. Pressure above 21 mmHg is considered abnormal. Damage, however, can occur at different pressures in different individuals. Some patients develop glaucomatous nerve damage at pressures below 21 mmHg, while others develop nerve damage only at very high pressures. Your eye specialist will tell you whether your pressure is normal for you as an individual.

5 / How common is glaucoma?

In Canada, glaucoma is one of the most common causes of blindness. For every person blinded by glaucoma, six others have lost useful vision in one eye. Approximately 200,000 Canadians have chronic open-angle glaucoma but only half of that number are aware of it. The other types of glaucoma are much less common. Ask your eye specialist to tell you what type of glaucoma you have.

6 / I see very well and do not wear glasses. How can I have glaucoma?

It is important to remember that glaucoma does not affect your central vision. Glaucoma affects side vision first, and only affects central vision very late in the disease. Therefore, glaucoma has no effect at all on your need to wear glasses.

7 / Does glaucoma cause blindness?

Yes, if untreated. That is why regular eye examinations are so important. If glaucoma is treated promptly, it can usually be controlled and vision can be saved.

8 / Can my children inherit glaucoma from me?

Yes, this is possible, although not always the case. Children whose parents have glaucoma should have annual eye examinations after the age of eighteen.

9 / Is glaucoma contagious?

No, it is not an infectious disease.

10 / Is glaucoma caused by stress?

No. Unlike blood pressure, eye pressure is relatively unaffected by stress.

11 / What is cupping of the optic nerve?

The optic nerve at the back of your eye carries all of the visual stimuli to the brain. The normal optic nerve looks a bit like a doughnut. It has a pale central area called the cup. The rim surrounds the cup and is the part of the nerve carrying the electrical impulses from the eye to the brain. In glaucoma the rim gets thinner and the pale cup area gets bigger. This process is known as cupping. If your doctor says your nerve is cupped, this means your nerve is damaged, with an enlarged central cup and thin rim (see figure 2, p. 52).

12 / My doctor says there is a hemorrhage on my nerve. What does this mean?

In glaucoma a small hemorrhage can, on occasion, be seen on the rim of the optic nerve. This hemorrhage indicates that the pressure is too high for the optic nerve. If a hemorrhage is found, your eye specialist will usually recommend lowering your pressure to a safer level with eye drops, laser treatment, or surgery.

13 / What are the risk factors for glaucoma?

Individuals who are more likely to be at risk are:

1) Over age fifty
2) Related to someone with glaucoma
3) Of African descent
4) Very short-sighted

Perhaps the most important of these is being related to someone with glaucoma. Glaucoma is unusual in people under the age of fifty. It is more common in patients with a strong family history and in those who are very short-sighted. In North America blacks are three times as likely to develop glaucoma as are whites of the same age. There is also a slight increase in glaucoma in patients who suffer from diabetes.

14 / Does glaucoma cause high blood pressure?

No. Having glaucoma will not increase your blood pressure.

15 / If my blood pressure is high, will my eye pressure be high?

Not necessarily. Although there is an indirect relationship between high blood pressure and glaucoma, patients under stress or who experience a sudden increase in blood pressure do not usually have high eye pressure.

16 / Does glaucoma produce eye strain and headaches?

No. Chronic glaucoma is symptomless. Most patients do not know they have the disease.

17 / Should I avoid over-the-counter medications if I have chronic glaucoma?

Over-the-counter medications should be avoided only if your eye specialist tells you that your angle is narrow; that is, that you are at risk of angle-closure glaucoma – an unusual form of glaucoma. Prescription drugs occasionally indicate on the package insert that they should not be used by patients with glaucoma. What is really meant is that patients at risk of angle-closure glaucoma should not use the medication as the drug may dilate the pupil, resulting in acute glaucoma. Ask your eye doctor to explain the type of glaucoma you have. Generally, patients with chronic glaucoma can use any prescription and non-prescription drug as none of these has adverse effects in relation to glaucoma. The exception is steroids, which, in both oral and eye-drop form, can aggravate chronic glaucoma.

18 / Some patients with glaucoma feel pain. Is this common?

Most patients who feel pain suffer from acute glaucoma, an unusual form of glaucoma. Patients may have loss of vision, severe pain, a red eye, nausea and vomiting, and very high intraocular pressure. Sometimes before the attack begins patients will see haloes around lights. This condition requires immediate eye-drop treatment, followed by laser treatment (see figure 3, p. 53)

19 / What is the cause of acute glaucoma?

Acute glaucoma is caused by the sudden closure of the drainage channels by the iris (the coloured part of the eye). This type of glaucoma is cured by laser treatment to the iris (see figure 3, p. 53).

20 / Does glaucoma cause cataracts?

There is no relationship whatsoever between glaucoma and cataracts. However, as glaucoma and cataracts both tend to occur in older patients, they often appear around the same time.

21 / Does caffeine make glaucoma worse?
Although some studies have indicated that caffeine has an effect on glaucoma, most of the recent studies suggest that drinking coffee and/or tea in moderation will not unduly influence your glaucoma.

22 / Will I go blind from glaucoma?
If diagnosed and treated early, glaucoma will not produce blindness. If diagnosed late, glaucoma which has gone untreated can cause permanent loss of vision.

23 / Can vision deteriorate despite treatment for glaucoma?
Yes. As we get older, we lose cells in the optic nerve responsible for vision. This is part of the normal aging process. Patients with severe damage from glaucoma will be more aware of this progressive loss of vision. At the present time there is very little that can be done about this change due to aging. It is therefore essential that glaucoma be diagnosed early before damage occurs to the nerve cells.

24 / Who diagnoses and treats glaucoma?
Glaucoma is usually discovered during a

routine eye examination performed by an optometrist or ophthalmologist. All ophthalmologists are trained to treat glaucoma with drugs, lasers, and surgery. Your eye specialist may refer you to a glaucoma specialist if there is doubt about the diagnosis or if there is need for further care.

25 / Will my glaucoma ever go away?

No. Glaucoma never goes away. The best we can do currently is to control glaucoma with eye drops, laser treatment, or surgery.

26 / Is any research being done to promote early diagnosis of glaucoma?

Yes. Much research is currently being done on the development of tests to enable us to diagnose damage at an earlier stage. These tests include colour-vision tests, flicker tests, contrast-sensitivity tests, and nerve-fibre-layer tests.

27 / Are there any popular misconceptions about glaucoma?

The majority of North Americans have the mistaken belief that vision lost to glaucoma can be restored. In a recent survey approximately 54 per cent of North Americans indicated that they believe that eye damage from glaucoma can be corrected. As well, 53 per cent reported that they believe that in the early stages of glaucoma, one can feel increased pressure in the eyes. Although these beliefs are common, they are mistaken.

28 / In the early stages of glaucoma can I feel pressure in my eye?

No. Glaucoma causes vision loss without warning symptoms.

29 / Does glaucoma commonly cause blindness in black North Americans?

Yes. Glaucoma is the most common cause of blindness in individuals of African origin. African–North Americans are at least three times as likely to develop glaucoma damage than are whites of the same age.

30 / Does emotional stress affect my intraocular pressure?

There is no scientific evidence to suggest that emotional stress affects intraocular pressure.

31 / Can lack of sleep or emotional stress associated with the visual field test push my pressure up on the day of the eye examination?

There is no evidence to suggest that lack of sleep the night before an examination or anxiety about the eye exam or the visual field test can change eye pressure.

32 / Will changing my diet or taking herbs help my glaucoma?

No. There is no evidence that changing one's diet will influence glaucoma. There is also no evidence that taking herbs (such as billberry) influences glaucoma.

33 / Does smoking or drinking alcohol have an impact on my glaucoma?

Neither alcohol use nor smoking causes glaucoma, although alcohol can lower intraocular pressure for a few hours under certain conditions.

34 / My eyes feel gritty and tender. Is this a result of the high pressure from glaucoma?

No. Chronic glaucoma has absolutely no symptoms at all. Grittiness is often caused by slightly dry eyes, a condition which can be made worse by overuse of eye drops.

35 / Will sexual activity affect my glaucoma?

No. Sexual activity has no positive or negative effect on glaucoma.

36 / Can babies be born with glaucoma?

Yes, babies can be born with or develop congenital glaucoma. This very rare form of glaucoma is characterized by tearing, enlargement of the front of the eye, and sensitivity to light. This condition is not related to the more common chronic open-angle glaucoma experienced by adults. Similarities, however, include an increase in pressure in the eye. In a baby this is due to poor development of the drainage system. Unlike the treatment of adult forms of glaucoma, treatment of congenital glaucoma is always surgical.

37 / How does chronic glaucoma differ from other glaucomas?

Chronic open-angle glaucoma is by far the most common form of glaucoma. It occurs in older patients and is due to poor drainage of fluid from the eye. There are, however, many other causes of glaucoma – all due to blockage of the drainage system in the angle of the eye. These rare forms of glaucoma can be caused by new vessels (seen in patients with diabetes or with blockage of a blood vessel in the eye), inflammatory material (seen in patients with a condition called uveitis or iritis), or pigment granules from the iris (seen in patients with pigmentary glaucoma, and also in those with a condition known as pseudoexfoliation). Trauma to the eyeball can also cause glaucoma by damaging the drainage system.

38 / Is eye pressure affected by menopause?

There is no evidence that menopause either raises or lowers eye pressure, or that menopause affects glaucoma.

39 / My distance vision has deteriorated a lot in the past few months. Is this due to glaucoma?

Glaucoma does not affect distance vision. Occasionally, however, Pilocarpine (an eye drop used to treat glaucoma) can make the pupil become so small that inadequate amounts of light get into the eye. This can lead to decreased vision, particularly in a dark room.

40 / My eyeball hurts when I read a lot. Does eye strain cause glaucoma?

No. Eye strain does not cause glaucoma.

41 / Can a blow to the eye cause glaucoma?

Trauma to the eye can lead to the development of glaucoma, when damage has been done to the drainage system (the trabecular meshwork). Rarely does one get glaucoma after a hard blow to the eye. If you have received a hard blow to the eye, though, you should be examined regularly to rule out the possible development of glaucoma, or, more commonly, retinal detachment.

42 / What is pseudoexfoliation?

Pseudoexfoliation is the shedding of a flaky white material found throughout the eye. It is best seen on the lens. Its presence is often associated with glaucoma. Patients with pseudoexfoliative glaucoma often have very high

eye pressure, which can be more difficult to
control. This type of glaucoma responds well
to the usual therapies, including laser trabeculoplasty.

43 / What is pigmentary glaucoma?

Pigmentary glaucoma is an unusual form of
glaucoma occurring in young, often short-
sighted adults. It is characterized by the presence of pigment granules throughout the eye,
which block the drainage system. Occasionally the pigment can cause blurred vision during vigorous exercise. As is the case in patients
suffering from pseudoexfoliation (see question 42), pressure is often high in the eyes of
those with pigmentary glaucoma. This type of
glaucoma responds well to the usual treatment, including laser treatment.

44 / What is neovascular glaucoma?

Neovascular glaucoma forms when new vessels in the angle of the eye block the drainage
system. These vessels are associated with a
number of conditions, including diabetes,
after blockage of a blood vessel at the back of
the eye (retinal vein occlusion), or when there
is poor blood supply to the eye. This type of
glaucoma is very difficult to control and is
treated with eye drops, oral medications, laser
treatment, and often eye surgery. Vision is
often poor in patients with this condition.

Tests for Glaucoma

1 / How often should I undergo testing for glaucoma?

If your glaucoma is well controlled, most ophthalmologists recommend twice-yearly eye exams.

2 / Are any of the tests for glaucoma painful?

No. The tests include a pressure test of the eyes, a field of vision test (which tests peripheral vision), and an eye examination.

3 / Why does my ophthalmologist use drops to enlarge my pupils? Can this damage my eyes?

Your ophthalmologist will dilate your pupils so that he or she can get a good look at the optic nerve at the back of the eyes. Careful examination of the optic nerve head will indicate to the ophthalmologist whether your glaucoma is well controlled. Although dilating drops cause blurred vision for up to forty-eight hours, the procedure will not in any way damage your eyes.

4 / Why does my ophthalmologist shine bright lights in my eye at every examination?

In order to diagnose glaucoma your eye specialist needs to examine the optic nerve thoroughly. To do this, he or she needs to shine lights into your eyes. Although the bright lights are uncomfortable they will not permanently affect your vision or damage your eyes.

5 / Is the visual field test bad for my eyes?

No. Although patients are expected to sit for at least fifteen to twenty minutes concentrating carefully on the visual field target, the test does not cause any damage to the eyes. The test itself may make the eyes feel tired but they soon recover with no permanent or long-term effects.

6 / Why must I have a visual field test so often?

The visual field test is an extremely important part of the eye examination for glaucoma. Glaucoma causes loss of side vision long before central vision becomes damaged, and the only way to test side vision is with the visual field test. Although this test is tiring for most patients, the results are very helpful in determining whether your glaucoma is under control. If your ophthalmologist notices a change in your vision during the visual field test you will be informed and your treatment will be adjusted accordingly.

7 / Does the field test cause discomfort?

In many cases, yes. Up to 30 per cent of the population experience difficulty with the test. It requires prolonged concentration without moving the eyes for up to twenty minutes at a time. Many patients find this test tiring. If you need to rest in the middle of the test you should mention this to the technician.

8 / What is a diurnal tension curve?

The diurnal tension curve shows changes in eye pressure. It is well known that intraocular pressure varies throughout the day. This variation is particularly marked in patients with glaucoma. It is possible that you could visit your eye doctor with a normal pressure at 4 p.m. but have a high pressure at 8 a.m. Therefore your eye doctor may ask you to stay a full day at the office and have your pressure checked every hour or two until the office closes. In university hospitals this test can often go on until late at night or early into the following morning. The test is very useful in determining your pressure profile. Treatment reassessment often depends on the results of the whole-day test.

9 / What methods are used to measure pressure?

The most common technique used to measure pressure involves the use of a machine called a tonometer. This small device is applied to your eye during a routine eye examination. You may notice a blue light very close to your eye. This blue-light test is used by the eye specialist to check your pressure.

10 / What is the yellow dye placed in my eye before a pressure test?

Fluorescein is a harmless dye that shows bright green in the presence of blue light. The application of fluorescein allows the eye specialist to accurately measure your pressure with the tonometer.

11 / I have undergone a procedure in which I'm told to lie flat while the specialist puts a metal device on my eye. What is the purpose of this?

This is a form of pressure testing called Schiötz tonometry. It is an older method of pressure testing, and has generally fallen into disuse.

12 / What other methods exist to check pressure?

There are a number of other methods to check pressure, including puff tonometry. A puff tonometer is a device that measures intraocular pressure after delivering a blast of air to the eye. Other pressure testing techniques include one which uses a small computerized penlike device to measure pressure. The blue-light test (see question 9) remains the 'gold standard' for pressure testing.

13 / I recently underwent scanning laser ophthalmoscopy. What is this?

The scanning laser ophthalmoscope is a relatively new device that uses a laser beam to scan the optic nerve. Early studies indicate that this device accurately measures the amount of damage to the optic nerve by measuring the size of the cup and the rim area (see question 11, section I, for further explanation). It is hoped that the scanning laser ophthalmoscope will eventually allow for very accurate measurement of early changes in the nerve at the back of the eye.

14 / Is the scanning laser ophthalmoscope dangerous?

No. The amount of light used during scanning laser ophthalmoscopy is much less than that used in standard eye photography. There is no evidence that scanning laser ophthalmoscopy in any way damages the eye.

15 / What are fundus photographs? Why do I need them?

Fundus photographs are taken to establish a baseline of optic nerve damage. At subsequent visits your eye doctor will compare the state of your optic nerves with the images on your photos. This will provide information as to whether your glaucoma is stable or not.

16 / Will the bright flashes of the photos damage my eyes?

No. Although the bright flashes may cause temporary discomfort, they will not damage your eyes.

All about Treatment

Eye Drops

1 / What if I forget to take my eye drops?

Take them as soon as you remember. In order to control your glaucoma, drops should be applied regularly, according to your doctor's instructions.

2 / What about side effects from drops? Can they be avoided?

Eye drops can adversely affect the lungs and heart in some circumstances. To prevent this keep your eyes closed for three minutes after instillation. It is recommended you push on the side of the nose where your upper and lower eyelids meet (applying this pressure is called nasolacrimal occlusion). This prevents drops from entering the nose through the tiny channels that drain tears from the eye. Nasolacrimal occlusion can prevent systemic absorption of drops by up to 40 per cent.

3 / I use three eye drops. How far apart should I space these drops?

It is not advisable to put your drops into your eye all at once. You should wait at least three to five minutes between drops. This prevents dilution and loss of drug in the form of tear-drops.

4 / Does it matter which drop goes in first?

If one of the drops you are taking is TIMOP-TIC XE®, it should go into your eye last.

5 / Do the eye drops cause cataracts?

Modern-day eye drops probably do not cause cataracts. However, some of the older eye drops, such as Phospholine Iodide, may pre-dispose patients to cataract formation. Eye doctors therefore tend not to use very strong drops such as Phospholine Iodide in patients who still have a normal lens.

6 / Can I miss the occasional eye drop?

No. Every time you forget to put an eye drop into your eye there will be no medication in the eye to control the pressure. Consequently, the pressure may increase causing further damage to your sight. Consistent self-treat-ment is an essential part of preventing blind-ness from glaucoma.

A / Miotics (Pilocarpine [Isopto® Carpine, Miocarpine™] Carbachol, Phospholine Iodide®)

7 / How do miotics work?

Miotics lower eye pressure by increasing the flow of fluid out of the drainage system located in the angle of the eye.

8 / If my vision is worse with a miotic drop does this mean I am allergic to this drop?

No. All miotics make the pupil small. This can lead to a decrease in vision because less light is allowed into the eye. This is an unavoidable side effect of Pilocarpine. If you experience this side effect, do not stop using your eye drop, but mention the change in your vision to your eye doctor.

9 / If my vision is worse with a miotic should I stop using it?

No. Unfortunately, miotics make your pupil small, which, as indicated above, can lead to a decrease in vision. However, Pilocarpine is very effective in lowering pressure in the eye, preventing damage from glaucoma. If your vision is worse with Pilocarpine continue to use the drop and mention this side effect to your eye doctor.

10 / What are the side effects of Pilocarpine and other miotic eye drops?

The common side effects from Pilocarpine and the other miotics include eye or brow pain, dim vision, blurriness of vision, and occasional redness of the eyes. Fortunately, however, most patients are able to tolerate these side effects. Very occasionally retinal damage may possibly occur. With retinal detachment the patient will typically see flashing lights and small dark floating spots. This may be followed by a curtain-like blocking of the vision. Patients experiencing these symptoms should stop using the drops and see their eye doctor immediately.

11 / Pilocarpine eye drops give me a headache. Should I stop using them?

No. Pilocarpine often initially produces severe eye discomfort. However, after a few days the pain settles down and usually goes away. In a small minority of patients, however, some mild pain continues. If the pain is very severe, simple analgesics usually control it. In most patients the pain will eventually disappear after a few days.

12 / Will I ever be able to stop using my drops?

No. Glaucoma never gets better. You should

never stop using your drops unless instructed
to do so by your eye doctor.

B / Beta Blockers (Timolol [TIMOPTIC®, TIMOPTIC XE®], Levobunolol [Betagan®], Betaxolol [Betoptic®])

13 / I use a beta blocker. What are they and how do they work?

These drugs inhibit the formation of eye fluid.
This decreased production leads to lower
intraocular pressure. There are many types of
beta blocker eye drops. They all work in a similar fashion by reducing the flow of the aqueous fluid into the eye. Examples of beta
blockers are Timolol, Levobunolol, and Betaxolol. Most are used twice a day. TIMOPTIC
XE® is used once a day.

14 / I have asthma. Can I use beta blockers?

No. Beta blocker eye drops should not be used
by patients with asthma as they can aggravate
this condition. Betaxolol has less effect on
lung function than do other beta blockers, but
it too can occasionally affect lung function,
especially in asthmatics.

15 / Do beta blockers produce any side effects?

Beta blockers such as Timolol usually produce
very few side effects. However, patients with

asthma and heart failure or heart block can find that these conditions are made worse by this group of drugs. In rare occasions beta blockers produce psychological problems such as depression, sleep disturbances, and impotence. Cold fingers and poor circulation are sometimes a problem. Betaxolol (Betoptic®) produces fewer heart and lung problems. However, this group of drugs should also be avoided by patients with heart failure or asthma.

16 / What is TIMPILO®?

TIMPILO® is a combination of Timolol and Pilocarpine. It is formulated in such a way as to allow for a twice-a-day dosage schedule. This combination does away with the need for drops three to four times a day. However, the shelf-life of the drug is short, and it should be replaced monthly. Timpilo is not available in all countries.

C / Adrenergic Agonists (Epinephrine [Eppy, Epitrate], Propine®)

17 / What are the side effects of Propine® and other adrenergic agonist eye drops?

Propine® and other epinephrine-like eye drops often cause the eye to become red with a slightly dilated pupil. More unusual side effects include raised blood pressure, angina, and excessive sweating.

18 / Do these drugs cause allergic reactions?

Allergic responses are common with these
drops. Often they initially cause the eye to
become whiter than usual, and then red a few
hours after instillation. Other side effects
include dilated pupils and rapid heart rate.

D / Oral Medications

19 / Can tablets such as Diamox® and Neptazane® help treat my glaucoma, and if so, how?

Tablets are definitely useful in treating glaucoma. Acetazolamide and Methazolamide
(Diamox® and Neptazane®) are commonly
prescribed for glaucoma. They effectively
lower the pressure in the eye by decreasing
the amount of eye fluid produced.

20 / Do tablets have any side effects?

As with all medications, tablets for the
treatment of glaucoma produce side effects.
Specific problems include upset stomach,
tingling in the fingers and toes, excessive
urination, feelings of depression or tired-
ness, loss of weight, formation of kidney
stones, and, very occasionally, failure of
the blood cells to mature (aplastic anemia),
a condition which can be fatal. Luckily,
however, this last side effect is extremely
rare.

E / Other Medications

21 / What is Apraclonidine (Iopidine®)?

Iopidine® is a relatively new drug which was initially used to prevent pressure increases after laser treatment. A drop of Iopidine® is inserted in the eye one hour before and one hour after laser treatment. The drop significantly prevents pressure spikes – large, sudden increases in pressure – in patients needing glaucoma laser surgery. More recently this drop has been shown to be effective both alone or in combination with the beta blockers used to treat glaucoma. As a result, this agent is now prescribed for long-term use in some patients with glaucoma.

22 / What are the side effects from Iopidine®?

Iopidine® commonly causes irritation and redness of the eye and allergic reactions. It can also produce nasal discomfort. Its effectiveness decreases over time in some patients.

23 / What is Dorzolamide (TRUSOPT®)?

Dorzolamide (TRUSOPT®) is a carbonic anhydrase inhibitor. It is applied in drop form to the eye and therefore does not cause many of the side effects associated with oral administration of these drugs (see question 20). This drug effectively lowers intraocular pressure, both when used alone or in combination with other eye drops. It should not be used in patients with known sulphonamide allergy. In theory it can result in failure of blood cells to mature (a condition known as aplastic anemia) but to date no such cases have been reported. This drop often stings when it is inserted, and it can produce an unpleasant taste in the mouth. An allergic reaction can also occur.

24 / Is smoking marijuana beneficial in relation to glaucoma?

Intraocular pressure can be lowered by smoking marijuana. Unfortunately, however, the effect is not long lasting. As a consequence one has to be constantly under the influence of marijuana to keep intraocular pressure under control. In view of the fact that marijuana is illegal, and as its effect on intraocular pressure is not prolonged, it should not be used to treat glaucoma. There are much better medications currently available for glaucoma therapy.

25 / Are there any new medicines being developed for glaucoma?

Yes. Carbonic anhydrase inhibitor drugs are available in some countries in eye-drop form for use in patients with glaucoma (see question 23). This means that patients currently taking Acetazolamide or Methazolamide (Diamox® or Neptazane®) may eventually be able to reduce their dosage or switch to the drop form. This should significantly decrease the incidence of side effects associated with the use of tablets (see question 20). Other potentially useful drugs for glaucoma include a group of drugs called the prostaglandins (e.g., Latanoprost). These drugs lower intraocular pressure, and are now available in Japan for this purpose. These latter drugs can change eye colour in some patients.

Laser Treatment

1 / What is laser trabeculoplasty?

Laser trabeculoplasty is the standard laser procedure performed on patients with chronic open-angle glaucoma. A laser beam is applied to the trabecular meshwork (the drainage portion located in the angle of the eye), usually in two sessions approximately one to two months apart (see figure 4, p. 54). The procedure is done while the patient is sitting at the slit lamp. It is painless, performed without a need for anaesthesia. It does, however, cause the patient to see bright flashes of light, and some patients complain of mild discomfort during the procedure.

2 / Does laser treatment cause cataracts?

There is no evidence that laser treatment causes cataracts.

3 / Will laser treatment cure my glaucoma?

Laser trabeculoplasty will not cure your glaucoma. In most cases it brings the eye pressure back under control by improving drainage of fluid from the eye. Recent statistics indicate that pressure in up to 50 per cent of the cases treated in this manner is still controlled five years after the procedure.

4 / What are the dangers of laser trabeculoplasty?

Laser trabeculoplasty is remarkably safe. However, eye pressure can sometimes increase suddenly after treatment. This increase in pressure can be controlled with the appropriate medications. Your eye specialist will usually ask you to stay at the office for at least an hour after the procedure to ensure that your pressure has not jumped to unacceptable levels. Other minor complications include mild visual disturbance for a few hours, and a slightly inflamed eye for a few days.

5 / Does Argon laser trabeculoplasty always work?

No. Argon laser trabeculoplasty has a high success rate during the first year after treatment. However, by the five-year mark only about 50 per cent of patients still have well-controlled pressures. This means there is a

50–50 chance that in five years the intraocular pressure will still be controlled.

6 / Do I need to continue using my drops after laser treatment?

Yes. After laser treatment patients are not usually allowed to stop using their eye drops. Laser therapy does, however, bring the uncontrolled pressure back within normal limits in patients on eye-drop treatment.

7 / Can laser treatment be used alone?

Yes. Patients who are allergic to or intolerant of drops or tablets can undergo laser treatment as a primary form of therapy. However, current opinion in North America still favours the use of eye drops first, followed by laser therapy if required.

8 / Why do I need laser treatment if my vision is good?

It is critical to understand that with glaucoma, central vision is not affected until very late in the disease.

9 / What is a laser iridotomy?

A laser iridotomy is a hole made in the coloured part of the eye (the iris). It is done to treat acute glaucoma or to prevent acute glaucoma from developing (see question 18, section I). It is also used to treat patients with other forms of angle-closure glaucoma (see figure 3, p. 53).

10 / Can laser iridotomy result in a hole that is too large? What are the other complications?

Laser iridotomy usually produces a very small hole. Occasionally the hole does allow extra light into the eye, resulting in the patient seeing a horizontal, slightly discoloured line that appears to move when he or she blinks. This visual disturbance is not serious but can be bothersome to some patients. It can be corrected with an appropriate contact lens but usually simple reassurance is all that is required to alleviate the symptom. Other rare complications include damage to the lens, retina, or cornea. Other complications include transient pressure spikes, slight bleeding from the iris, and mild inflammation of the eye. These latter three complications respond well to appropriate therapy and cause no long-term problems.

11 / How long should I stay home from work after laser treatment?

Laser treatment (both iridotomy and trabeculoplasty) should not affect your ability to work. Usually you can go back to work the day after the procedure. Very occasionally, laser treatment can produce inflammation, which may make the eye uncomfortable. In this situation you may have to stay home from work for a couple of days.

12 / I have been told I need a ciliary body destructive procedure. What is this?

Destruction of the ciliary body (a procedure called cycloablation) is done either with a laser beam, or with a cryoprobe (a freezing device). It is a treatment used only on eyes where the intraocular pressure is uncontrolled despite conventional treatment. Transscleral cyclocoagulation (done with a laser) is currently the procedure of choice to treat patients with severe glaucoma. The procedure is done under local anaesthetic. It takes approximately ten minutes, and has a success rate of approximately 65 per cent. Complications include loss of some vision in some patients, pain and discomfort, a red eye for a few weeks, excessively low pressure, and hemorrhaging. In view of these complications this procedure is performed only in cases where blindness is a significant risk. Freezing treatment (cyclocryotherapy) achieves similar results but is associated with more complications, and is therefore used less often than laser treatment. It is most commonly used on blind, painful eyes with high pressure, but can be very effective in other select cases.

Surgery

1 / What kind of surgical treatment is available for glaucoma? How successful is it?

Filtration surgery, which creates a new drainage system from within the eye to under the lining membrane of the eye (conjunctiva), is called trabeculectomy (see figures 5 and 6, pp. 55 and 56). The surgery is done under local anaesthesia and takes approximately three-quarters of an hour to perform. It is done using an operating microscope. This surgery has a success rate of approximately 75–90 per cent. Some people, however, do need to continue to use eye drops after surgery. Unfortunately, approximately 10 per cent of the patients require more than one operation to bring the pressure under control. Very occasionally, the surgery can actually cause vision loss, but this occurs in less than 5 per cent of the patients.

2 / Does glaucoma surgery cause cataracts?

There is some evidence to suggest that patients who undergo glaucoma surgery may have a slightly increased tendency to form cataracts. As previously discussed, loss of sight from cataracts can be surgically treated. Loss of sight from glaucoma, however, is irreversible.

3 / Do I need to stay in hospital if I have glaucoma surgery?

In North America, patients are usually treated as out-patients; that is, their surgery is done under local anaesthetic and they are allowed to go home a few hours later. Patients are, of course, advised to go straight to bed and not to bend over or physically exert themselves for at least twenty-four to forty-eight hours.

4 / Is surgery painful?

Most surgeries are performed under local anaesthetic. This means that you will be awake and you will feel a few pinpricks at the start of the operation. During the operation you will feel pulling sensations but no pain. You can talk to your surgeon if required, but silence is generally preferred.

5 / What happens if I attempt to blink during surgery?

You may feel the need to blink during surgery. A special lid instrument called a speculum will be placed between your eyelids to ensure that they remain open during the whole procedure. Blinking will therefore in no way affect your surgery.

6 / What happens if I cough during surgery?

Slight movements and gentle coughs are not usually a problem during surgery. Severe coughing, however, can be disruptive to the surgeon and make surgery difficult to perform.

7 / Can I see during the operation?

The eye not being operated on will be covered during the surgery. The eye being operated on will be prepared and cleaned with antiseptic, and then the local anaesthetic will be administered. Some local anaesthetics cause loss of vision while others do not. Ask your surgeon which type of local anaesthetic is to be used in your case. If it is the latter, you will see a bright light with moving shadows during the operation.

8 / Will my eye hurt after surgery?

Once the local anaesthetic wears off you may feel some pain, especially when moving the eye or blinking. If this occurs simply keep both eyelids closed and take a painkiller. Most patients do not need one, but do check with your family practitioner before surgery regarding the appropriate painkiller for you. Severe eye pain is most unusual after glaucoma surgery; if you do experience severe pain you should contact your eye surgeon for further advice.

9 / What can go wrong during eye surgery?

Trabeculectomy has been the standard operation for glaucoma for over twenty years, and it is generally a safe, effective procedure. However, complications occasionally occur. They can include injury from the local anaesthetic injection (very rare) and intraocular bleeding. Mild bleeding is usually not a problem for the patient or surgeon. It can, however, lead to prolonged rehabilitation. Sudden bursting of a blood vessel in the eye during or after surgery causes severe pain and is an extremely rare complication that can lead to permanent vision loss. Other surgical difficulties can occasionally occur. They can all be dealt with by a competent surgeon, but may prolong the recovery a little.

10 / What are antifibroblastic agents?

Antifibroblastic agents are drugs that are used to prevent closing of the surgical wound, and thereby improve the chances of successful surgery. However, they are associated with some complications and are not routinely used. They are used on patients requiring repeat surgery or who have complicated glaucomas. There are two drugs in this family:

5-Fluorouracil (5-FU). This anticancer drug effectively improves surgical success, especially in patients who have previously had unsuccessful surgery, or in patients who have previously had cataract surgery. The drug can be applied during surgery, or administered daily via injections to the surface of the eye for a period of three to ten days. Complications from the drug include corneal ulcers and eye discomfort. Corneal ulcers sometimes develop on the front of the eye after four or more treatments. These ulcers can be painful but usually settle down within a few weeks after treatment with drops and the wearing of an eye patch. Mild eye discomfort may result from daily injections.

Mitomycin. This anticancer drug is an effective antihealing agent. It is applied during surgery to the surgical site. It is more convenient for both patient and surgeon than 5-FU because of its intraoperative use. Complications, however, can be more serious than with 5-FU. This drug is so effective that it can produce excessive drainage of fluid through the newly created surgical site. The low pressure that can result is known as hypotony and can be associated with a larger than usual bleb (see question 23) and a soft eye. A soft eye, that is, one with pressure below 4 mmHg, may result in decreased vision. If the eye remains excessively soft over a long period of time it can be treated with injections of blood into the wound area, or can be surgically repaired. A large thin bleb can occasionally become infected, necessitating antibiotic therapy to the eye.

11 / Is there a role for early surgery in glaucoma?

There is no doubt that there is a trend towards earlier surgery these days. Evidence from Europe indicates that patients undergoing early surgery may do better over the long term. There are of course complications associated with surgery, and as a consequence ophthalmic surgeons in North America still recommend drops first, followed by laser treatment and surgery only as a last resort. However, this line of approach seems to be slowly changing.

12 / What is successful surgery?

Surgery is successful when the pressure in the eye is reduced by about 30 per cent, whether the patient is on or off medication. The key to success is a reduction in pressure to a level that prevents ongoing nerve and visual field damage.

13 / What can go wrong after surgery?

Although the success rate for surgery is high (75–90 per cent), complications occasionally occur. These include:

1) Postoperative complications such as a soft eye (called a flat anterior chamber) due to excessive drainage of fluid from the eye (see question 19). This usually heals with appropriate care in five to seven days but does occa-

sionally require surgical intervention to remedy the excessive drainage.

2) Blurred vision for up to six weeks.

3) In rare instances, total loss of vision. It is not clearly understood why this occurs but it does seem to happen in patients with very severe vision loss before the glaucoma surgery. Other complications include infection, hemorrhaging, damage to the eye or the optic nerve from the local anaesthetic injection, discomfort, change in refraction (strength of glasses), droopy lid, and development of ciliary block glaucoma (see question 22).

14 / How will my eye look after surgery?

Immediately after surgery your eye will be bloodshot and swollen. However, over a four-to-six-week period it will whiten and should eventually look virtually normal. Occasionally, however, the eyelid may droop a little or you may see a white blob appear from under the upper lid (see question 23).

15 / My eye feels dry after surgery. Is this normal?

It is not uncommon for a patient's eye to feel gritty and dry after surgery. This is usually because the tear film is not spread evenly over the front of the eye. Should this occur it is important to avoid dry environments like air-conditioned cars. Topical lubricants can often relieve this symptom.

16 / My eye feels wet since surgery. Is this normal?

Occasionally after surgery the wound may leak for a few weeks. This usually causes slight dampness, particularly during the night, and on awakening. This symptom should be reported to your eye surgeon. There are a number of ways to cure such leaks, including the use of eye patches, topical drops, contact lens, and, occasionally, surgical repair of the leak. Leaks usually resolve spontaneously.

17 / The doctor massaged my eye after surgery. Is this a routine procedure?

It is common for the eye surgeon to massage the eye after surgery. The purpose of this procedure is to push fluid through the little hole created during the operation. In fact, your eye surgeon may teach you how to massage your own eye. The massage keeps the surgical wound open, keeping the pressure in the eye low. Do not massage your eye unless instructed by your eye surgeon. Initially massage may be uncomfortable, especially if done a day or two after surgery. However, it will not damage the eye if performed by an eye surgeon, or by yourself as directed by your surgeon.

18 / Can high pressure develop after surgery?

High eye pressure after surgery usually means that the new surgical passage is partially blocked. This can be dealt with by eye massage (see question 17) and laser burns to stitches (suture lysis) (see question 20).

19 / Can surgery produce a soft eye?

The purpose of the surgery is to allow eye fluid (the aqueous humour) to leave the eye through a covered hole (2 mm × 2 mm) created by your surgeon. On occasion excessive leakage can occur during the early postoperative period. This can lead to a soft eye with a flat anterior chamber. Your surgeon will determine the extent of the overfiltration and may recommend the following:

(a) An eye patch. A simple eye patch plus drops usually resolves the problem in three to ten days.

(b) Glue or a contact lens over the leaky area, with or without a patch. In addition, eye drops are prescribed.

(c) Surgical repair. If the drainage is excessive it may be necessary to insert air or fluid into the eye to 'pump up' the eye a little. Occasionally choroidals are drained after surgery to help re-form the eye. Choroidals are fluid-filled cystlike areas that develop in the eye when the pressure is very low. Sometimes surgeons place an extra stitch or two into the surface of the eye (conjunctiva or sclera) to stop a leak.

20 / My surgeon says I need a suture cut after glaucoma surgery. Is this necessary?

After surgery you may need to have a stitch cut to help bring the pressure under control. Cutting a suture is painless for the patient and easy to do with the laser. It does not require a scalpel blade. It is usually done under topical anaesthesia, that is, with the use of an eye drop and a special contact lens. The procedure usually takes no more than a couple of minutes. It is commonly followed by eye massage (see question 17).

21 / Can surgery cause blindness?

Glaucoma surgery is usually very successful (see question 1). It is possible, however, that some patients may lose vision after surgery. This is extremely rare and usually occurs only in patients with very severe glaucomatous damage at the time of surgery.

22 / My doctor says I have malignant glaucoma (ciliary block). What is this?

Ciliary block glaucoma can develop after surgery, and is characterized by high pressure. The cause of this pressure is a fluid imbalance between the back and the front of the eye. In this condition the fluid passes towards the back of the eye instead of through the normal chambers in the front of the eye. This complication has absolutely nothing to do with cancer. Today the condition is reversible, with the use of eye drops and oral medications, in 50 per cent of the cases. The other 50 per cent require further surgery to remedy the condition.

23 / Since surgery I have noticed a raised white blob under my upper lid. What causes this?

After glaucoma surgery, fluid flows out of the eye under a thin membrane called the conjunctiva. When this membrane swells and is filled with fluid it produces a small balloonlike structure under the upper eyelid called a bleb, which can be seen by lifting the upper lid. It is not a cause for concern. In fact, it is a good sign, as it means the operation has been effective (see figure 6, p. 56).

24 / Do blebs become less effective with time?

Blebs do shrink with time and can scar up. When this happens, the pressure will increase, eventually leading to the reintroduction of the use of eye drops, and possibly repeat surgery.

25 / Can blebs cause problems?

Large blebs in themselves can produce a number of symptoms including discomfort and irritation. Large blebs can and do push on the eye and cause astigmatism. A change in eyeglass prescription may therefore be required after surgery.

26 / Can blebs cause discomfort?

A dry area occasionally develops in front of the bleb, causing discomfort and some pain. This is readily relieved by using artificial tears to wet the dry area.

27 / My bleb is still present but my pressure is increasing. Is this a problem?

Blebs do become less effective with time for two reasons: (1) glaucoma often gets worse with age; (2) blebs tend to scar. If your pressure starts increasing the ophthalmologist will initially recommend restarting medical therapy, which usually controls the situation. If not, repeat surgery is always an option.

28 / Can blebs have serious complications?

Yes. Blebs very occasionally become infected and/or leak spontaneously. Leaks can occur after excessive trauma to the eye. Leaks can cause low pressure, resulting in blurry vision, and can make the eye susceptible to infection. Infection can be caused by swimming in contaminated water, or from poor lid hygiene. Infections are extremely rare but serious.

29 / How do I know if my bleb is infected?

A bleb infection is characterized by a mild to moderate yellow or green discharge, a very red eye, blurry vision, and a white bleb. This is an ocular emergency requiring admission to hospital and intensive treatment with antibiotics. If the infection is caught early the eye will be saved. The bleb, however, may scar or leak after an infection.

30 / Should I take any precautions after my surgery?

Glaucoma surgery is based on the principle of making a new drainage system in the eye. Any excessive exercise or trauma for the first weeks can lead to softening of the eye and damage. It is important not to exert oneself excessively for the first two to three weeks following surgery. Sexual activity is permissible after this time period.

31 / My doctor says I need a molteno implant. What is this?

A molteno implant is one of a number of plastic tubelike devices (called Setons) inserted into the eye to help drainage of fluid from the eye to the tissues surrounding the eye (see figure 7, p. 57). A seton implant is performed only when conventional surgery has failed because of scarring. The tube bypasses the scarred part of the eye, causing the pressure to come under control. Technically this is a more involved operation than a simple trabeculectomy. Successful control of pressure is often possible, but the complication rate is higher. Complications include damage to the cornea, erosion of the tube, high intraocular pressure postoperatively, low intraocular pressure postoperatively, damage to the lens, pain and discomfort for the patient, and double vision. Despite these complications, the success rate for molteno implants is rather good. Furthermore, they can save sight in eyes that might otherwise be doomed to blindness.

Glaucoma Societies

1 / In Canada
The Glaucoma Research Society of Ontario is an organization run by members of the public which depends on charitable donations to help fund research at academic institutions. Their address is 1 Spadina Cres., Toronto, Ontario M5S 2J5. Their telephone number is (416) 978-2635.

2 / In the United States
In the United States the Foundation for Glaucoma Research, at 490 Post St., Ste. 830, San Francisco, CA 94102–1409, supports glaucoma research.

3 / In the United Kingdom
In the United Kingdom the International Glaucoma Society, at Kings College Hospital, London, U.K. SE5 9RS, supports research and education on glaucoma.

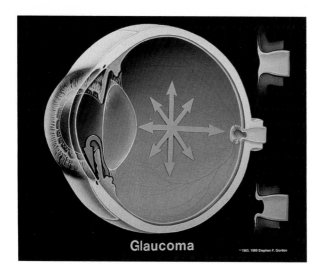

Glaucoma

Figure 1: Flow of fluid through the eye. Obstruction to flow in the front of the eye (green arrows) increases pressure in the eye (blue arrows) leading to damage to the optic nerve at the back of the eye. The depressed area in the middle of the optic nerve is the result of an abnormal process called cupping.

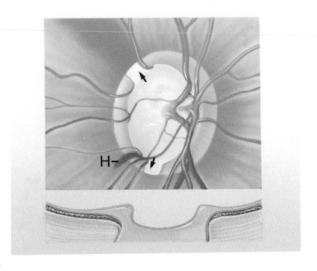

Figure 2: Nerve damage in glaucoma. The central white area is known as the cup. The arrows show areas of damage (notches) on the rim of the nerve. 'H' is a hemorrhage on the rim of the nerve. Hemorrhages, notches, and cupping occur if the pressure in the eye is at an unacceptable level. The bottom of the picture shows a severely cupped nerve.

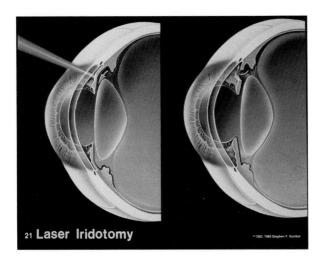

21 **Laser Iridotomy**

Figure 3: Effect of a laser burn (iridotomy) on the iris after treatment of acute glaucoma. The arrow shows the unimpeded passage of fluid through the hole created by the laser burn.

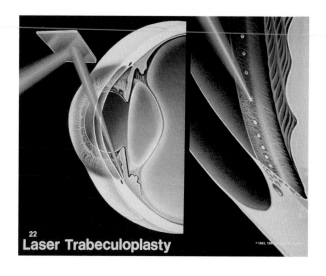

Figure 4: Laser trabeculoplasty. The laser is focused through a mirror into the trabecular meshwork in the angle of the eye. The white spots show the heating effect caused by the laser.

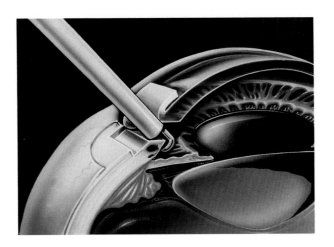

Figure 5: Filtration surgery. Note the creation of a
channel to allow the fluid to leave the eye.

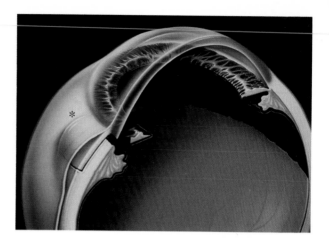

Figure 6: This shows the end result of a trabeculectomy surgical procedure. A trap door covered by a
membrane called a bleb (see asterisk) allows the fluid
to leave the eye.

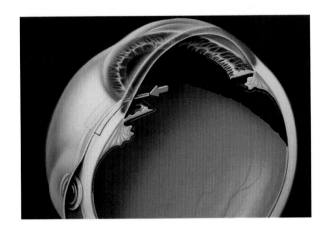

Figure 7: A seton (molteno implant). The blue arrow
indicates the passage of fluid from inside the eye to a
base plate well away from both the potential area of
scarring and the scarred surgical site.

Glossary of Glaucoma Terms

adrenergic agonists. A class of eye drops related to epinephrine that reduces eye pressure by decreasing production and increasing outflow of aqueous humour.

angle-closure glaucoma. An unusual and painful form of glaucoma requiring emergency medical and laser treatment.

antifibroblastic agents. Anticancer drugs used to prevent scarring after glaucoma surgery.

aplastic anemia. A potentially lethal form of blood thinning occasionally caused by carbonic anhydrase inhibitors.

aqueous humour. The interior eye fluid produced by the ciliary processes. This fluid nourishes the front of the eye and drains out through the trabecular meshwork. Eye pressure is modified by changes in production or drainage of this fluid.

beta blockers. The most commonly used class of glaucoma eye drops. Beta blockers inhibit the formation of aqueous humour, thereby lowering intraocular pressure. They can precipitate asthma and heart failure in susceptible individuals.

bleb. A raised swelling usually found under the upper eyelid after successful glaucoma surgery. It is formed by aqueous humour collecting under the conjunctiva.

carbonic anhydrase inhibitors. A class of drugs used either topically (e.g., TRUSOPT®) or orally (e.g., Diamox®) to decrease intraocular pressure by inhibiting aqueous production. These drugs are related to the sulfonamides.

choroidal effusion. Choroidals are fluid-filled cyst-like areas formed at the back of the eye, usually within the first few weeks after glaucoma surgery, when the pressure is very low. They resolve as eye pressure increases. They are occasionally drained surgically to relieve a flat chamber.

chronic open-angle glaucoma. The most common form of glaucoma, occurring in over 90 per cent of all patients with glaucoma. Also known as primary open-angle glaucoma.

ciliary block glaucoma. A very rare form of glaucoma that develops after glaucoma surgery. It is also called malignant glaucoma. It has nothing to do with cancer, and responds well to medical and/or surgical treatment.

ciliary body destructive procedure. The destruction of the ciliary body in order to decrease the production of aqueous humour and thereby lower pressure. This can be achieved by utilizing a freezing device (cryoprobe) or a laser (laser cyclocoagulation).

ciliary processes. Small finger-like organs found in the eye, responsible for the production of aqueous humour.

conjunctiva. The thin transparent membrane lining the sclera of the eye. It forms the lining of the bleb after a trabeculectomy.

cupping. An abnormal process that occurs within the optic nerve, often in association with high pressure. Cupping is associated with loss of nerve tissue in the optic nerve, leading to visual field loss.

diurnal tension curve. A test to determine the variation of intraocular pressure throughout the day. This variation is exaggerated in patients with glaucoma. Testing the pressure every one to two hours often allows for diagnosis of raised pressure.

flat chamber. A fairly common problem occurring after glaucoma surgery. It is due to excessive drainage of aqueous humour from the eye and is often associated with the formation of choroidal detachments. This condition is characterized by low eye pressure and contact between the iris and the cornea, and usually resolves with appropriate medical therapy. Surgical intervention is occasionally required.

fluorescein. A yellow-orange nontoxic dye that shines brightly in the presence of a special blue light. Fluorescein is placed in the eye before pressure is measured during tonometry.

fundus photographs. Photographs taken of the optic nerve head as a baseline measure of the amount of cupping for future comparison.

glaucoma. Characteristic optic nerve and visual field loss often associated with raised pressure. The most common form is chronic or primary open-angle glaucoma.

glaucoma suspect. An individual with high intraocular pressure but without nerve cupping or visual field damage. A glaucoma suspect is also referred to as being ocular hypertensive.

hypotony. A situation where the eye is very soft. It develops after surgery and can be associated with a decrease in vision.

iritis. Inflammation of the coloured part of the eye (the iris). Also known as uveitis.

laser iridotomy. A procedure performed to prevent or cure angle-closure glaucoma.

laser trabeculoplasty. A laser procedure performed to lower intraocular pressure in patients with chronic open-angle glaucoma.

low-pressure glaucoma. An unusual form of glaucoma in which there is characteristic glaucoma nerve damage and visual field loss but a normal intraocular pressure. It is treated in the same way as chronic open-angle glaucoma.

malignant glaucoma. *See* ciliary block glaucoma.

miotics. A class of drugs that improve the flow of aqueous humour out of the eye. Miotics cause the pupil to become small, sometimes resulting in decreased vision. Headaches are a common side effect of these drugs.

molteno implant. One of the many different types of setons used after failed glaucoma surgery. It consists of a long tube inserted into the eye. The tube is attached to a base plate, which is stitched onto the sclera.

nasolacrimal occlusion. The application of pressure to the corner of the eye where two eyelids meet at the side of the nose. After application of drops, three minutes of nasolacrimal occlusion while keeping the eyelids closed will reduce systemic absorption of medication by up to 40 per cent. This will substantially reduce side effects, especially on the heart and lungs.

neovascular glaucoma. A rare form of glaucoma in which small blood vessels grow and cover the trabecular meshwork. Diabetes and retinal vein occlusion are the most common causes of this condition. This form of glaucoma is difficult to treat and is often associated with poor vision in the affected eye.

ocular hypertension. *See* glaucoma suspect.

optic nerve. The nerve that connects the back of the eye to the brain. Damage to this nerve is the cause of vision loss in glaucoma.

pigmentary glaucoma. An unusual form of glaucoma occurring in younger patients who are often mildly short-sighted. The iris releases pigment, which accumulates on various structures of the eye, including the trabecular meshwork. This form of glaucoma responds well to standard therapy and particularly to laser treatment.

primary open-angle glaucoma. *See* chronic open-angle glaucoma.

pseudoexfoliation. A form of glaucoma fairly common in older individuals, characterized by dandruff-like flakes of white material accumulating on various structures in the eye. The pressure is often high in patients with pseudoexfoliation, and this form of glaucoma often needs aggressive treatment. It responds well to the usual therapies, including laser treatment.

retinal vein occlusion. A blood clot in one of the small blood vessels at the back of the eye. Retinal vein occlusion can occur in patients with uncontrolled glaucoma. It can also cause a rare form of glaucoma called neovascular glaucoma.

scanning laser ophthalmoscopy. A relatively new form of imaging which uses a laser beam to capture three-dimensional images of the optic nerve head.

Schiötz tonometry. An older form of tonometry in which a metal device is placed on the eye while the patient is lying down.

sclera. The white, opaque outer lining of the eye, through which a trabeculectomy incision is made during glaucoma surgery.

sulfonamides. The class of drug to which the carbonic anhydrase inhibitors belong. Patients with sulfonamide allergies should not use these agents.

suture lysis. A laser procedure performed after trabeculectomy in which a scleral stitch is cut to allow for improved flow of aqueous humour from the eye.

Successful suture lysis leads to improved bleb formation and lower intraocular pressure.

tonometer. A special device applied to the eye, commonly associated with a bright blue light, used to measure intraocular pressure. Glaucoma is usually diagnosed and monitored with Goldmann tonometry.

trabecular meshwork. The drainage system of the eye that becomes blocked in glaucoma.

trabeculectomy. The most commonly used surgical procedure to lower intraocular pressure in patients with glaucoma.

transscleral cyclocoagulation. A laser procedure used to destroy the ciliary processes in patients with glaucoma.

uveitis. *See* iritis.

visual field. The range of peripheral and central vision, tested to both diagnose and monitor visual function in patients with glaucoma.

visual field test. A specialized vision test used to check the visual field of a patient with glaucoma. Computerized methods are used in most glaucoma centres. Humphrey, Octopus, and Dicon Perimeters are the pieces of equipment most widely used to test the visual field.